Vegetarian R
Everyc

Incredible Tasty Meals to Start ·our vcyctaiiaii way and Lose Weight

America Best Recipes

Table of Contents

Breakfast
Milky Scrambled Tofu
Preparation Time: 10 minutes Cooking time: 10 minutes

Servings: 4

Ingredients:

7 ounces almond milk

2 tablespoons flax meal mixed with 2 tablespoons water

2 tablespoons firm tofu, crumbled

Cooking spray

Salt and black pepper to the taste

8 cherry tomatoes, cut into halves

Directions:

In a bowl, mix flax meal with milk, salt and pepper and whisk well.

Grease your air fryer with cooking spray, pour flax meal, add tofu, cook at 350 degrees F for 6 minutes, scramble them a bit and transfer to plates.

Divide tomatoes on top and serve. Enjoy!

Breakfast Bell Peppers

Preparation Time: 10 minutes Cooking time: 10 minutes

Servings: 8

Ingredients:

1 yellow bell pepper, halved

1 orange bell pepper, halved

Salt and black pepper to the taste

ounces firm tofu, crumbled

1 green onion, chopped 2 tablespoons oregano, chopped

Directions:

In a bowl, mix tofu with onion, salt, pepper and oregano and stir well. Place bell pepper halves in your air fryer's basket and cook at 400 degrees F for 10 minutes. Leave bell pepper halves to cool down, peel, divide tofu mix on each piece, roll, arrange plates, and serve right away for breakfast. Enjoy!

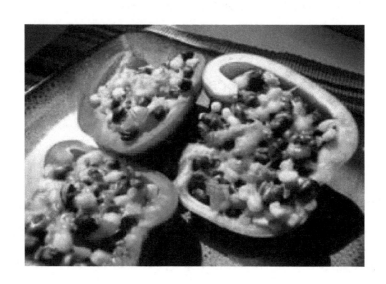

French Toast Pudding

Preparation time: 5 minutes Cooking time: 0 minutes

Servings: 5

Ingredients:

4 Bananas, Chopped

1 Cup Almond Milk

2 Tablespoons Maple Syrup

4 Slices Vegan French Bread

1 Teaspoon Vanilla Extract, Pure

1 Tablespoon Almond Butter

¼ Teaspoon Ground Cloves

1 Teaspoon Cinnamon 1 Cup Water

Directions:

Pour in your water, and then get out a round pan. Chop the bread and place it on the bottom.

Blend your maple syrup, chopped bananas, vanilla extract, cloves and cinnamon together until smooth, pouring it into the pan with the bread.

Cover the pan with foil and make sure the edges are secure. Transfer it into the instant pot and then close your lid.

Cook on high for sixteen minutes on the pudding setting. Use a quick release, and then add your almond butter in, and stir gently before serving.

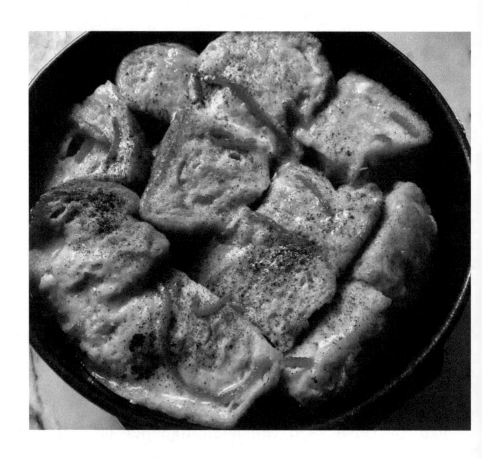

Morning Forest Maple Granola

Preparation time: 5 minutes Cooking time: 20 minutes

Servings: 4 ½ cups.

Ingredients:

2 cups oats 1/3 cup pumpkin seeds

1/3 cup sunflower seeds

1/3 cup walnuts

1/3 cup unsweetened coconut flakes

¼ cup wheat germ

1 ½ tsp. cinnamon

1 cup raisins

1/3 cup maple syrup

Directions:

Begin by preheating the oven to 325 degrees Fahrenheit. Next, mix all of the above ingredients—except for the raisins and the maple syrup—together in a large bowl. After you've mixed the ingredients well, add the maple syrup, and thoroughly coat the other ingredients.

Next, spread out this mixture on a baking sheet and bake the granola for twenty minutes, making sure to stir every four minutes or so.

After twenty minutes, add the raisins and bake for an additional five minutes. Remove the baking sheet and allow the granola to cool for forty-five minutes. Enjoy!

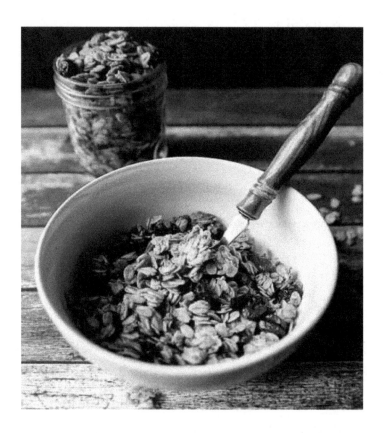

Silky Whole Wheat Strawberry Pancakes

Preparation time: 5 minutes Cooking time: 25 minutes

Servings: 24 pancakes.

Ingredients:

1 ¾ cup whole wheat flour

1/3 cup cornmeal

½ tsp. baking soda

1 tsp. baking powder

½ tsp. cinnamon

2 tbsp. maple syrup

2 cups vanilla soymilk

4 cups sliced strawberries

Directions:

Begin by combining all the dry ingredients in a mixing bowl. Stir well, and create a hole in the center of the mixture to pour the syrup and soymilk into it.

Continue to stir, making sure not to over-stir. Next, add half of the strawberries into the mixture. Heat the skillet or the griddle, and portion just a bit of Earth Balance butter overtop.

Drop little pieces of the batter onto the skillet and cook both sides of the pancakes. Keep the pancakes warm as you cook the batter's remainder and top the pancakes with strawberries. Enjoy.

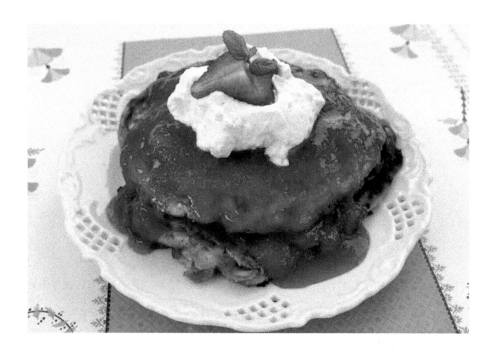

Apple and Cream Instant Pot Quinoa

Prep time: 10 min Cooking Time: 6 min Serve: 2

Ingredients

½ cup quinoa

1 cup of water

1 1/2 cups coconut milk

1/8 teaspoon salt

1/8 teaspoon ground nutmeg

2 tablespoons maple syrup

½ cup apple

Instructions

Add the ingredients to the Instant Pot, stirring the mixture together.

Lock lid.

Let it cook and naturally release.

When the quinoa has finished cooking, serve and enjoy!

Nutrition Facts

Calories514, Total Fat 31.4g, Saturated Fat 25.7g, Cholesterol 0mg,Sodium 173mg, Total Carbohydrat 55.1g, Dietary Fiber 7g, , Total Sugars 21.8g , Protein 8.9g

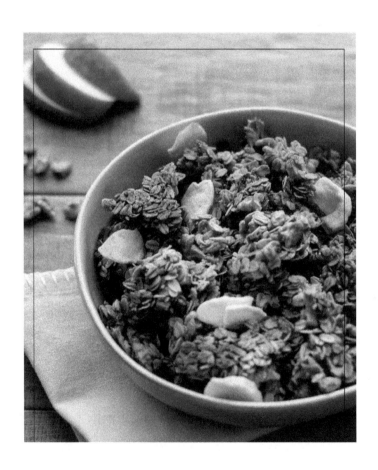

Breakfast Cobbler

Prep time: 10 min Cooking Time: 15 min Serve: 2

Ingredients

1 peach, diced

1 apple, diced

½ cup blueberries

2 tablespoons honey

1 tablespoon coconut oil

¼ teaspoon ground nutmeg

¼ cup unsweetened shredded coconut

2 tablespoons sunflower seeds

Instructions

Place your cut fruits into the stainless steel bowl of your Instant Pot. Spoon in the honey and coconut oil, sprinkle the nutmeg, lock lid.

Press the Steam button; the display will read 10 minutes. Allow the fruit to cook, and quickly release the pressure once the cooking cycle has completed. Remove the lid once safe to transfer the cooked fruit with a slotted spoon or skimmer into a serving bowl.

Now place the coconut, and sunflower seeds into the residual liquid and press the Sauté button.

Allow the contents to cook, shifting them regularly so they do not burn. Once they are nicely browned and toasted, about 5 minutes or so, remove them.

Serve!

Nutrition Facts

Calories284, Total Fat 12.3g, Saturated Fat 9g, Cholesterol 0mg, Sodium 4mg, Total Carbohydrate 47.2g, Dietary Fiber 6g , Total Sugars 40.2g, Protein 2.3g

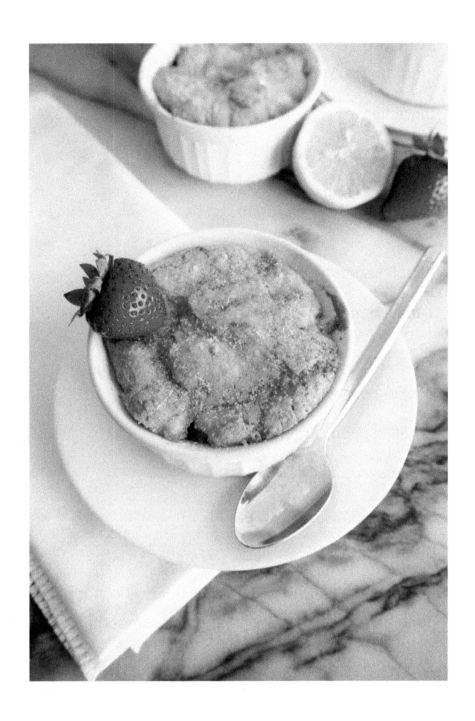

Pancake

Prep time: 05 min Cooking Time: 45 min Serve: 2

Ingredients

1 cup coconut flour

½ cup coconut milk

1 egg

1 tablespoon honey

1 teaspoon baking powder

½ teaspoon salt

Cooking spray

½ tablespoon butter, for serving

Maple syrup, for serving

Instructions

In a large bowl, mix all coconut flour, coconut milk, egg, honey, baking powder and salt until smooth.

Using non-stick cooking spray, grease the bottom and sides of Instant Pot. Pour batter into Instant Pot and lock lid. Set to Low Pressure. Cook for 45 minutes.

Use a spatula to remove pancake from pot. Serve with butter and maple syrup.

Nutrition Facts

Calories 139, Total Fat 9.5g, Saturated Fat 7.9g, Cholesterol 41mg, Sodium 331mg, Total Carbohydrate 11.7g, Dietary Fiber 3.8g, Total Sugars 6g, Protein 3.3g

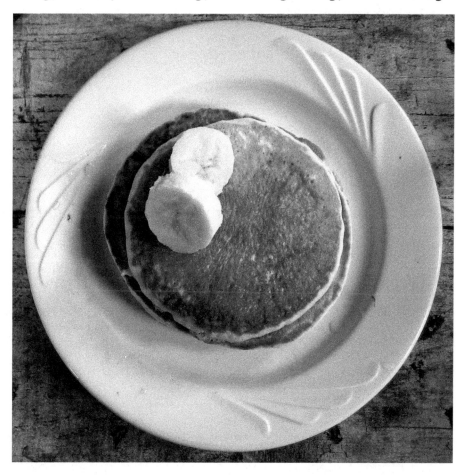

Swiss Chard Muffin

Prep time: 6 min Cooking Time: 10 min Serve: 2

Ingredients

2 eggs

1/8 teaspoon pepper seasoning

4 tablespoons shredded goat cheese

1 green onion, diced

½ cup Swiss chard chopped

1 1/2 cups water

Instructions

Put the steamer basket in the Instant Pot and add 2 cups of water.

Break eggs into a large measuring bowl with pour spout, add pepper, and beat well. Divide the cheese, Swiss chard and green onion evenly between muffin cups. Pour the beaten eggs into each muffin cup and stir with a fork to combine.

Place muffin cups on steamer basket. Cover and lock lid in place. Select High Pressure and 8 minutes cook time.

When timer beeps, turn off, wait two minutes, then use a quick pressure release.

Carefully open the lid, lift out the steamer basket, and remove muffin cups.

Serve immediately.

Nutrition Facts

Calories 66, Total Fat 4.7g, Saturated Fat 2.4g, Cholesterol 89mg , Sodium 66mg, Total Carbohydrate 0.8g, Dietary Fiber 0.2g , Total Sugars 0.5g, Protein 5.1g

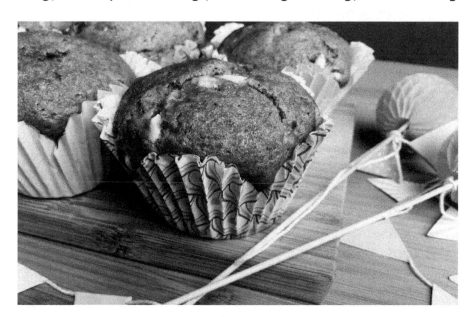

Tofu, Sweet Potato and Spinach Bowl

Prep time: 10 min Cooking Time: 10 min Serve: 2

Ingredients

Sweet Potato Layer

1 cup Sweet potatoes, cut into quarters

1½ cups water

Tofu Layer

¼ cup water

1 tablespoon honey

1 teaspoons soy sauce

½ teaspoon hot sauce, to taste

½ cup tofu , cut into small cubes

Spinach Layer

2 cups chopped spinach

1 tablespoon water

½ teaspoon garlic powder

Lunch
Baked Smoky Broccoli and Garlic

Ingredients

Cooking spray

1 tablespoon extra virgin olive oil

3 cloves garlic, minced

1/2 teaspoon sea salt

1/4 teaspoon ground black pepper

½ tsp. cumin

½ tsp. annatto seeds

3 1/2 cups sliced broccoli

1 lime, cut into wedges

1 tablespoon chopped fresh cilantro

Directions:

Preheat your oven to 450 degrees F. Line a baking sheet with foil and grease with olive oil. Mix the olive oil, garlic, cumin, annatto seeds, salt, and pepper in a bowl. Add in the cauliflower, carrots, and broccoli.

Combine until well coated. Spread them out in a single layer on the baking sheet. Add the lime wedges. Roast in the oven until vegetables become caramelized for about 25 minutes. Take out the lime wedges and top with the cilantro.

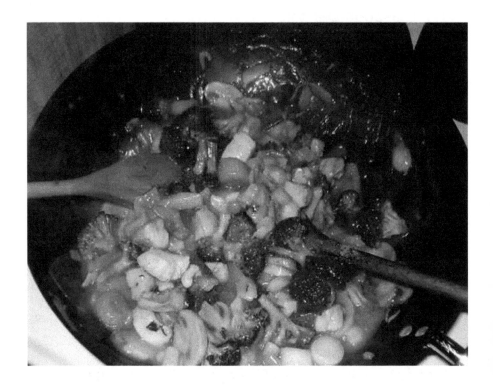

Asian Roasted Broccoli and Choy Sum

Ingredients

cooking spray

1 tablespoon sesame seed oil

3 cloves garlic, minced

1/2 teaspoon sea salt

1/4 teaspoon ground black pepper

3 1/2 cups sliced choy sum (Chinese Flowering Cabbage)

2 1/2 cups slice broccoli

1 tablespoon chopped fresh cilantro

Directions:

Preheat your oven to 450 degrees F. Line a baking sheet with foil and grease with olive oil. Mix the sesame oil, garlic, salt, and pepper in a bowl. Add in the choy sum and broccoli Combine until well coated. Spread them out in a single layer on the baking sheet. Roast in the oven until vegetables become caramelized for about 25 minutes. Top with the cilantro.

Roasted Cauliflower and Lima Beans

Ingredients

1 tablespoon melted vegan butter/margarine

9 cloves garlic, minced

1/2 teaspoon sea salt

1/4 teaspoon ground black pepper

1 1/2 cups sliced cauliflower

3 1/2 cups cherry tomatoes

1 (15 ounces) can lima beans, drained

1 lemon, cut into wedges

Directions:

Preheat your oven to 450 degrees F. Line a baking sheet with foil and grease with melted vegan butter or margarine. Mix the olive oil, garlic, salt, and pepper in a bowl. Add in the cauliflower, tomatoes, and lima beans. Combine until well coated. Spread them out in a single layer on the baking sheet. Add the lemon wedges.Roast in the oven until vegetables become caramelized for about 25 minutes. Take out the lemon wedges.

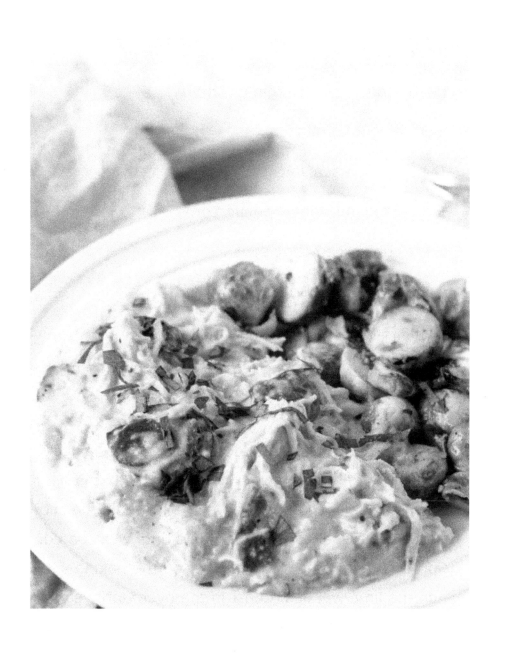

Roasted Brussel Sprouts and Choy Sum

Ingredients

1 tablespoon extra virgin olive oil

8 cloves garlic, minced

1/2 teaspoon sea salt

1/4 teaspoon rainbow peppercorns

3 1/2 cups sliced choy sum

2 1/2 cups sliced Brussels sprouts

1 lime, cut into wedges

1 tablespoon chopped fresh cilantro

Directions:

Preheat your oven to 450 degrees F. Line a baking sheet with foil and grease with olive oil. Mix the olive oil, garlic, salt, and pepper in a bowl. Add in the choy sum and Brussel sprouts. Combine until well coated. Spread them out in a single layer on the baking sheet. Add the lime wedges. Roast in the oven until vegetables become caramelized for about 25 minutes. Take out the lime wedges and top with the cilantro.

Thai Roasted Spicy Black Beans and Choy Sum

Ingredients

cooking spray

1 tablespoon sesame oil

3 cloves garlic, minced

1/2 teaspoon sea salt

1 tbsp. Thai chili paste

1/4 teaspoon ground black pepper

3 1/2 cups Choy Sum, coarsely chopped

2 1/2 cups cherry tomatoes

1 (15 ounces) can black beans, drained

1 lime, cut into wedges

1 tablespoon chopped fresh cilantro

Directions:

Preheat your oven to 450 degrees F. Line a baking sheet with foil and grease with sesame oil. Mix the olive oil, garlic, salt, Thai chili paste, and pepper in a bowl.

Add in the choy sum, tomatoes, and black beans. Combine until well coated. Spread them out in a single layer on the baking sheet. Add the lime wedges. Roast in the oven until vegetables become caramelized for about 25 minutes. Take out the lime wedges and top with the cilantro.

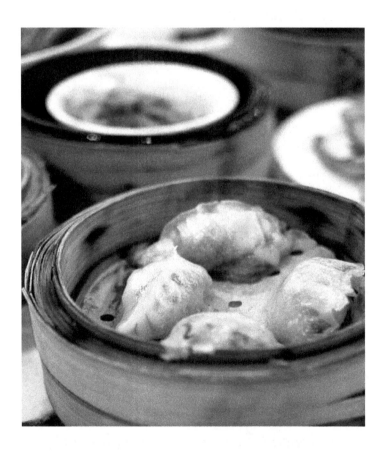

Roasted Red Potatoes and Asparagus

Ingredients

1 1/2 pounds red potatoes, cut into chunks

2 tablespoons extra virgin olive oil

12 cloves garlic, thinly sliced

1 tbsp. and 1 tsp. dried rosemary

4 teaspoons dried thyme

2 teaspoons sea salt

1 bunch fresh asparagus, trimmed and cut into 1 inch pieces

Directions:

Preheat your oven to 425 degrees F. In a baking pan, combine the first 5 ingredients and 1/2 of the sea salt. Cover with foil. Bake 20 minutes in the oven. Combine the asparagus, oil, and salt. Cover, and cook for about 15 minutes, or until the potatoes become tender. Increase your oven temperature to 450 degrees F. Take

out the foil, and cook for 8 minutes until potatoes become lightly browned.

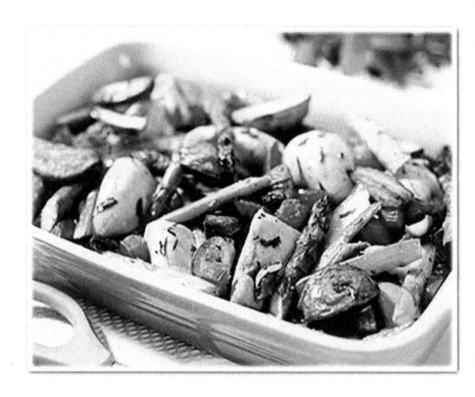

Baked Parsnips and Green Beans

Ingredients

1 1/2 pounds parsnips, cut into chunks

2 tablespoons extra virgin olive oil

12 cloves garlic, thinly sliced

1 tsp. Italian seasoning

4 teaspoons dried thyme

2 teaspoons sea salt

1 bunch green beans, trimmed and cut into 1 inch
pieces

Directions:

Preheat your oven to 425 degrees F. In a baking pan,
combine the first 5 ingredients and 1/2 of the sea salt.
Cover with foil. Bake 20 minutes in the oven. Combine
the green beans, oil, and salt. Cover, and cook for
about 15 minutes, or until the parsnips become tender.
Increase your oven temperature to 450 degrees F. Take

out the foil, and cook for 8 minutes until potatoes become lightly browned.

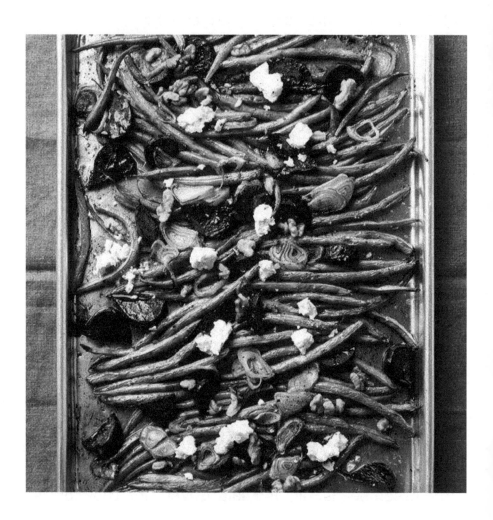

Roasted Lime Garlic Buttered Green Beans

Ingredients

1 1/2 pounds potatoes, cut into chunks

4 tablespoons butter

12 cloves garlic, thinly sliced

2 tsp. lime juice

2 teaspoons sea salt

1 bunch fresh green beans, trimmed and cut into 1 inch pieces

Directions:

Preheat your oven to 425 degrees F. In a baking pan, combine the first 5 ingredients and 1/2 of the sea salt. Cover with foil. Bake 20 minutes in the oven. Combine the green beans, oil, and salt. Cover, and cook for about 15 minutes, or until the potatoes become tender. Increase your oven temperature to 450 degrees F. Take out the foil, and cook for 8 minutes until potatoes become lightly browned.

Roasted Parsnips and Edamame Beans

Ingredients

1 1/2 pounds parsnips, cut into chunks

2 tablespoons extra virgin olive oil

12 cloves garlic, thinly sliced

1 tbsp. dried rosemary

4 teaspoons dried thyme

2 teaspoons sea salt

1 bunch edamame beans, trimmed and cut into 1 inch pieces

Directions:

Preheat your oven to 425 degrees F. In a baking pan, combine the first 5 ingredients and 1/2 of the sea salt. Cover with foil. Bake 20 minutes in the oven. Combine the edamame beans, oil, and salt. Cover, and cook for about

15 minutes, or until the turnips become tender. Increase your oven temperature to 450 degrees F. Take

out the foil, and cook for 8 minutes until potatoes become lightly browned.

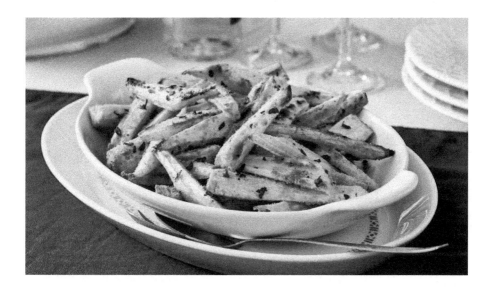

Roasted Escarole and Hearts of Palm

Ingredients

1 1/2 pounds escarole, cut into chunks

3 tablespoons extra virgin olive oil

12 cloves garlic, thinly sliced

1 tbsp. and 1 tsp. dried rosemary

4 teaspoons dried thyme

2 teaspoons sea salt

1 bunch hearts of palm, trimmed and cut into 1 inch pieces

Directions:

Preheat your oven to 425 degrees F. In a baking pan, combine the first 5 ingredients and 1/2 of the sea salt. Cover with foil. Bake 20 minutes in the oven. Combine the hearts of palm, oil, and salt. Cover, and cook for about 15 minutes or until the escarole becomes tender. Increase your oven temperature to 450 degrees F. Take out the foil, and cook for 8 minutes until potatoes become lightly browned.

Soups and Salads

Cottage Cheese Soup
(Prep time: 10 min| Cooking Time: 35 min| Serve: 2)

Ingredients

1 stalks leek, diced

1 tablespoon bell pepper, diced

¼ cup Swiss chard, sliced into strips

1/8 cup fresh kale

1 eggplant

½ tablespoon avocado oil

1/8 cup button mushrooms, diced

1 small onion, diced

½ cup cottage cheese

2 cups vegetable broth

1 bay leaf

½ teaspoon salt

¼ teaspoon garlic, minced

1/8 teaspoon paprika

Instructions

Place leek, bell pepper, Swiss chard, eggplant, and kale into a medium bowl, set aside in a separate medium bowl. Press the Sauté button and add the avocado oil to Instant Pot. Once the oil is hot, add mushrooms and onion. Sauté for 4–6 minutes until onion is translucent and fragrant. Add leek, bell pepper, Swiss chard, and kale to Instant Pot. Cook for additional 4 minutes. Press the Cancel button. Add diced cottage cheese, broth, bay leaf, and seasonings to Instant Pot. Click lid closed. Press the Soup button and set the time for 20 minutes. When the timer beeps, allow a 10-minute natural release and quickly release the remaining pressure. Add eggplant on Keep Warm mode and cook for additional 10 minutes or until tender. Serve warm.

Nutrition Facts:

Calories 212, Total Fat 3.6g, Saturated Fat 1.2g, Cholesterol 5mg, Sodium 1603mg, Total Carbohydrate 30.7g, Dietary Fiber 11.9g, Total Sugars 12.7g, Protein 17g

Cauliflower Soup
(Prep time: 10 min| Cooking Time: 5 min| Serve: 2)

Ingredients

5 cups vegetable broth or water

1 medium onion chopped

1 - 2 stalks leek thinly sliced

2 cloves garlic crushed

1 lb. cauliflower cut in big chunks

1 teaspoon salt

1/2 teaspoon pepper

1 teaspoon fresh basil

1/4 cup almond flour

2/3 cup water

1 cup grated goat cheese

1/2 cup milk

Salt and pepper to taste

Instructions

Add the first 8 ingredients (including basil) to the Instant Pot and lock lid. Make sure the valve is set to Sealing and press Pressure Cooker (or Manual). Set the time with the + /- button for 5 minutes. While cooking, stir in flour and water until smooth. When the IP beeps, flip the valve from Sealing to Venting, and when the pin drops, press Cancel and remove the lid. Press the Sauté button and cook again, stirring frequently. Whisk the flour-water mixture and add about half of it to the soup. Use a hand blender to puree the soup. Or use a blender or food processor and put it back in the pan. Press Cancel and add the cheese. Stir until melted. Do not cook after the cheese has gone in. Add the milk, salt, and pepper to your taste. Serve with a pinch of grated cheese.

Nutrition Facts

Calories 202, Total Fat 8.4g, Saturated Fat 4.4g, Cholesterol 20mg, Sodium 1345mg, Total Carbohydrate 23.2g, Dietary Fiber 7.8g, Total Sugars 11.3g, Protein 12.6g

Pumpkin Soup

(Prep time: 10 min| Cooking Time: 20 min| Serve: 2)

Ingredients

1 lb pumpkin peeled and seeded 1/2-1-inch cubes

1 cup vegetable broth or water

1 teaspoon dried rosemary

1/4 teaspoon grated cinnamon

1/2 teaspoon salt

1 cup coconut milk

2 tablespoons butter

1 tablespoon almond flour

Instructions

Mix the pumpkin cubes, broth, rosemary, cinnamon, and salt in an Instant Pot. Lock the lid onto the pot.

Press Soup/Broth, Pressure Cooker, or Manual on High Pressure for 5 minutes with the Keep Warm setting off. The valve must be closed. Use the Quick-release mode to return the pot pressure to normal. Unlock the lid and open the pot. Add coconut milk.

Use an immersion blender to puree the soup right in the pot. Or work in halves to puree the soup in a covered blender. If necessary, pour all the soup back into the pan. Press the Sauté button and set it for Low, 250°F. Set the timer for 5 minutes. Bring the soup to a simmer, stirring often. In the meantime, place the butter in a small bowl or measuring container and place it in the microwave in 5-second increments. Use a fork to mix the flour and make a thin paste. When the soup is boiling, Whisk the butter mixture into the pan. Continue whisking until the soup is a bit thick, about 1 minute. Turn off the Sauté function and allow it to cool for a few minutes before serving.

Nutrition Facts

Calories 415, Total Fat 41g, Saturated Fat 32.9g, Cholesterol 31mg, Sodium 1064mg, Total Carbohydrate 11.5g, Dietary Fiber 3.3g, Total Sugars 5.2g, Protein 5.9g

Vegetarian Spinach Soup
(Prep time: 15 min| Cooking Time: 20 min| Serve: 2)

Ingredients

½ tablespoon coconut oil

¼ onion, finely chopped

½ stalk leek, finely chopped

1 teaspoon garlic powder

1 teaspoon basil, freshly chopped

¼ teaspoon red pepper flakes (optional)

Salt

Freshly ground black pepper

2 cups vegetable broth

Enough water

1 (15.5oz.) can chickpea, drained and rinsed

Juice of 1 lemon

1 large bunch of Spinach, removed from stems and torn into medium pieces

Instructions

In an Instant Pot, press the Sauté button and set it for Medium, heat oil. Add onion, leek, and cook until slightly soft, 6 minutes. Add garlic powder, basil, and red pepper flakes and cook until fragrant, 1 minute more. Season with salt and pepper.

Add broth, water, lemon juice, chickpea, and Spinach. Press Soup/Broth, Pressure Cooker, or Manual on High Pressure for 10 minutes with the Keep Warm setting off. The valve must be closed. Use the Quick-release method to return the pot pressure to normal. Unlock the lid and open the pot.

Use an immersion blender to puree the soup right in the pot. Press the Sauté button and set it for Low, 250°F. Set the timer for 5 minutes.

Bring the soup to a simmer, stirring often.

Serve.

Nutritions:

50.7g, Dietary Fiber 15.2g, Total Sugars 9.8g, Protein 20.1g

Green Soup

(Prep time: 10 min| Cooking Time: 35 min| Serve: 2)

Ingredients

4 cups vegetable broth

1 small onion, cut into 3/4-inch pieces

1/3 cup rice

1 tablespoon vegetable oil

1 teaspoon garlic powder

Salt

1/4 cup Greek yogurt

1 tsp minced fresh mint

1/4 tsp finely grated lime zest plus 1/2 tsp juice

6 oz. collard greens stemmed and chopped

4 oz spinach, stemmed and chopped

1 cup beet greens

Instructions

Add broth, onion, rice, oil, garlic powder, and 1/2 teaspoon salt to a blender. Lock lid in place, the particular Soup program 2 (for creamy soups).

In the meantime, combine Greek yogurt, mint, lime zest, and juice, and remaining 1/4 teaspoon salt in a bowl; refrigerate until ready to serve. Pause program 12 minutes before it has been completed. Carefully remove the lid and stir in collard greens and spinach until wholly submerged. Return lid and resume program. Pause the program 1 minute before it has been completed. Stir in beet greens.

Return lid and resume program. Once the program has completed, adjust soup consistency with extra broth as needed and season with salt and pepper to taste. Drizzle individual portions with yogurt sauce before serving.

Nutrition Facts

Calories 306, Total Fat 9.7g, Saturated Fat 1.8g, Cholesterol 1mg 0%, Sodium 225mg, Total Carbohydrate 48.7g, Dietary Fiber 12.6g, Total Sugars 3.4g, Protein 13.6g

Crunchy Lemon Barley and Broccoli Bowl

(Prep time: 15 min| Cooking Time: 15 min | serve: 2)

Ingredients

½ cup fresh broccoli

1 teaspoon olive oil

½ onion, diced

½ teaspoon garlic powder

½ cup barley

¼ cup vegetable stock

½ tablespoon turmeric powder

½ lemon, juiced

¼ teaspoon kosher salt

Instructions

Pour the barley into the Instant Pot. Add the vegetable stock and kosher salt. Lock the lid into place. Select Pressure Cook or Manual, and adjust the pressure to

High and the time to 5 minutes. After cooking, let the pressure release naturally for 2 minutes, then quickly release any remaining pressure. Unlock the lid. Keep a side. Select Sauté in Instant Pot, add olive oil when it hot. Add the onion and garlic powder; cook until the onion is translucent, about 2 minutes. Stir in cooked barley and turmeric powder; cook until flavors combine for 5-6 minutes. Stir in broccoli and lemon juice; cook and stir 3-4 minutes. Serve and enjoy.

Nutrition Facts

Calories 225, Total Fat 3.7g, Saturated Fat 0.6g, Cholesterol 0mg, Sodium 22mg, Total Carbohydrate 41g, Dietary Fiber 10g, Total Sugars 2.6g, Protein 7.1g

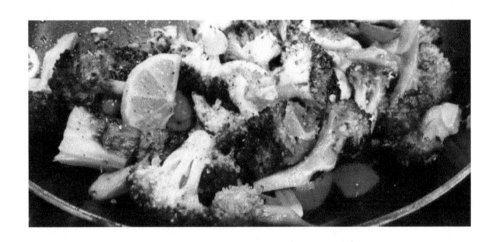

Strawberry Millet Salad

(Prep time: 15 min| Cooking Time: 10 min | serve: 2)

Ingredients

¼ cup millet

1 cup water

1 teaspoon lemon juice

1 teaspoon coconut oil

2 cups baby kale, or to taste

2 cups almonds

½ cup goat cheese, crumbled

½ cup thinly sliced strawberries, or to taste

Instructions

Pour the millet into the Instant Pot. Add the water and Lock the lid into place. Select Pressure Cook or Manual, and adjust the pressure to High and the time to 10 minutes. After cooking, let the pressure release naturally for 2 minutes, then quickly release any remaining pressure. Unlock the lid. Combine lemon juice and coconut oil in a small bowl; stir until dressing is combined. Pour half of the millet into a large salad bowl. Add 1 handful of baby kale; stir together. Add 1 handful of almonds, goat cheese, and strawberries; stir until mixed. Repeat layering and stirring barley, kale, goat cheese, and strawberries until all ingredients are mixed. Top with the dressing.

Nutrition Facts

Calories 774, Total Fat 53.7g, Saturated Fat 7.5g, Cholesterol 7mg, Sodium 49mg, Total Carbohydrate

46g, Dietary Fiber 15.7g, Total Sugars 6g, Protein 26.8g

Green Apple and Pecans Salad with Quinoa

(Prep time: 15 min| Cooking Time: 15 min | serve: 2)

Ingredients

1 cup water

½ cup quinoa

¼ cup pecans

½ cup diced green apple

1 diced cucumber

¼ cup diced red bell pepper

1/8 cup diced leek

Lemon, juiced

½ green onion, thinly sliced

1 teaspoon garlic powder

¼ teaspoon flaked salt

Instructions

Turn Instant Pot to Normal Sauté. Add oil and let heat for 1-2 minutes. Add pecans, often stirring, until toasted 2 minutes. Keep aside. Pour the quinoa into the Instant Pot. Add the water and lock the lid into place. Select Pressure Cook or Manual, and adjust the pressure to High and the time to 10 minutes. After cooking, let the pressure release naturally for 2 minutes, then quickly release any remaining pressure. Unlock the lid.

Combine quinoa, pecans, apples, cucumbers, red bell peppers, leeks, lemon juice, green onions, garlic powder, and salt in a bowl.

Nutrition Facts

Calories 257, Total Fat 4.3g, Saturated Fat 0.5g, Cholesterol 0mg, Sodium 12mg, Total Carbohydrate

46.6g, Dietary Fiber 6.6g, Total Sugars 10.5g, Protein 8.2g

Egg Salad

(Prep time: 15 min| Cooking Time: 5 min | serve: 2)

Ingredients

4 eggs

1 cup water

¼ cup chopped cucumbers

¼ cup carrots, chopped

1 tablespoon lemon juice and zest

1 tablespoon mustard

salt and ground black pepper to taste

Instructions

Pour the water into the Instant Pot. Place a steamer basket or the trivet in the pot. Carefully arrange eggs in the steamer basket. Secure the lid on the pot. Close the pressure-release valve. For hard-cooked eggs, select Manual and Cook at Low Pressure for 5 minutes. When cooking time is complete, use a Natural Release to depressurize. Remove the lid from the pot and gently place eggs in a bowl of cool water.

Combine eggs, cucumbers, carrots, lemon juice and zest, mustard, salt, and black pepper in a bowl.

Nutrition Facts

Calories 163, Total Fat 10.5g, Saturated Fat 2.8g, Cholesterol 327mg, Sodium 125mg, Total Carbohydrate 5.9g, Dietary Fiber 1.7g, Total Sugars 2.1g, Protein 12.9g

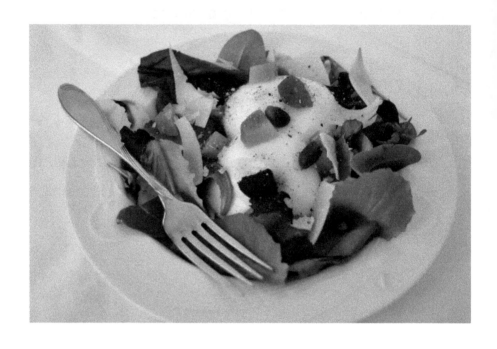

Magical Egg Salad

(Prep time: 15 min| Cooking Time: 10 min | serve: 2)

Ingredients

5 eggs

2 tablespoons Greek yogurt

2 tablespoons Dijon mustard

2 tablespoons carrots

¼ teaspoon red chili

¼ teaspoon dried rosemary

Salt and ground black pepper to taste

1 pinch cayenne pepper

Instructions

Pour the water into the Instant Pot. Place a steamer basket or the trivet in the pot. Carefully arrange eggs in the steamer basket. Secure the lid on the pot. Close the pressure-release valve. For hard-cooked eggs, select

Manual and Cook at Low Pressure for 5 minutes. When cooking time is complete, use a Natural Release to depressurize. Remove the lid from the pot and gently place eggs in a bowl of cool water. Chop eggs and transfer to a large bowl.

Stir Greek yogurt, Dijon mustard, carrots, red chili, rosemary into eggs until well mixed; season with salt and black pepper. Cover and refrigerate until chilled, if desired.

Sprinkle with cayenne pepper before serving.

Nutrition Facts

Calories 249, Total Fat 13.6g, Saturated Fat 5g, Cholesterol 414mg, Sodium 369mg, Total Carbohydrate 6.9g, Dietary Fiber 0.8g, Total Sugars 5.4g, Protein 24.8g

Dinner

Cottage cheese and Potato Coconut Curry

(Prep time: 10 min |Cooking Time: 10 min | serve: 2)

Ingredients:

1 package cottage cheese

1 cup vegetable broth

1 cup onion sliced

¼ teaspoon ginger powder

1/8 teaspoon turmeric powder

½ teaspoon cumin

1 cup potatoes, diced

1 cup coconut milk, unsweetened

Salt to taste

Pepper to taste

Instructions

1. In an Instant Pot, heat about 1/4 cup of the vegetable broth on Medium to high heat. 2. Add onions, ginger, turmeric, and cumin, and sauté. Add potatoes and sauté for a few minutes. 3. Crumble cottage cheese into tiny pieces (Resembling ground meat), mix well, and then add coconut

Milk. Close the Instant Pot, and using the Manual function, set the cooker to Low Pressure for 4 minutes.

When time is up, then quickly release. Remove the lid and, uncovered, simmer until liquid is absorbed. Add salt and pepper. Enjoy.

Nutrition Facts

Calories 233, Total Fat 5.2g, Saturated Fat 3.6g, Cholesterol 9mg, Sodium 930mg, Total Carbohydrate

26.4g, Dietary Fiber 3g, Total Sugars 3.7g, Protein 20.4g

Rutabagas Curry

(Prep time: 10 min |Cooking Time: 20 min | serve: 2)

Ingredients

4 rutabagas, peeled and cored from the top

1 tablespoon vegetable oil

½ onion, finely chopped

1 teaspoon ginger powder

1 teaspoon garlic powder

1 red tomato, pureed

¼ teaspoon turmeric

¼ tablespoon red chili powder

¼ teaspoon Garam masala

½ teaspoon salt

5 almonds

1/8 cup milk warm

½ tablespoon dried fenugreek leaves

Basil leaves

Instructions

Soak almonds in warm milk for 10 minutes and set aside. Set Instant Pot to Sauté mode. Once the ―Hot‖ sign displays, add vegetable oil. Add onions and cook for 2 minutes with a glass lid on, stirring few times. Add ginger and garlic powder, cook for 30 seconds. Add the carved-out pieces from the rutabagas. Add tomato paste, turmeric, red chili powder, Garam masala, and salt. Cook everything on Sauté mode for 2 minutes with a glass lid on, stirring a couple of times. With a small spoon, carefully fill the rutabagas with the cooked masala/gravy and line them all in the Instant Pot insert. Add 1/2 cup of water. Close the Instant Pot, using the Manual function, set the cooker to High Pressure for 8 minutes. When time is up, quickly release the pressure.

Blend milk and almonds to make a smooth paste. Stir in dried fenugreek leaves, almond paste, and chopped basil.

Set Instant Pot to Sauté mode, mix everything. Add salt to taste. Bring to a gentle boil, and then turn Instant Pot off. Serve with hot and. Enjoy!

Nutrition Facts

Calories 219, Total Fat 9.4g, Saturated Fat 1.7g, Cholesterol 1mg, Sodium 664mg, Total Carbohydrate 31g, Dietary Fiber 9.3g, Total Sugars 18.7g, Protein 6.2g

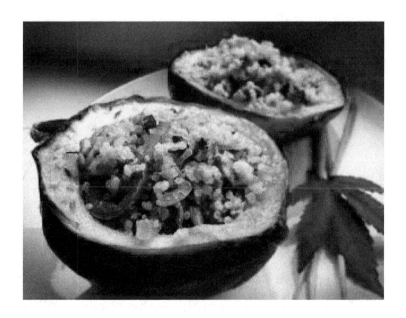

Spice-Rubbed Broccoli Steaks

(Prep time: 10 min |Cooking Time: 5 min | serve: 2)

Ingredients

1 small head of broccoli

1 tablespoon coconut oil

1 teaspoon red chili powder

1 teaspoon ground cumin

½ teaspoon salt

½ cup parsley fresh, chopped

½ lemon

Instructions

Insert the steam rack into the Instant Pot. Add 1½ cups water. Remove the leaves from the broccoli and trim the core, so the broccoli sits flat. Place on the steam rack. In a small bowl, combine the coconut oil, red chili powder, cumin, and salt. Drizzle over the broccoli and rub to coat.

Lock the lid. Using the Manual function, set the cooker to High Pressure for 4 minutes. Use the ―Quick Release‖ method to vent the steam, then open the lid.

Lift the broccoli onto a cutting board and slice into 1-inch thick steaks. Divide among plates and sprinkle with the parsley. Serve with lemon quarters. Enjoy!

Nutrition Facts

Calories 78, Total Fat 7g, Saturated Fat 5.9g, Cholesterol 0mg, Sodium 597mg, Total Carbohydrate

4.4g, Dietary Fiber 1.6g, Total Sugars 1.1g, Protein 1.4g

Spicy Eggplant

(Prep time: 10 min |Cooking Time: 15 min | serve: 2)

Ingredients:

1 tablespoon coconut oil

2 eggplants, cut into 1-inch cubes

1 onion, thinly sliced

½ tablespoon garlic powder

1 tablespoon soy sauce

1 cup water

1 teaspoon honey

Ground black pepper to taste

Salt to taste

Instructions

Set Instant Pot to Sauté mode, heat coconut oil. Cook and stir the eggplant cubes until they begin to brown about 3-5 minutes. Remove the eggplant with a slotted spoon, and set it aside. 2. Then add onions just until they begin to soften for about 30 seconds. Stir in the garlic powder, and cook and stir for an additional 30 seconds. Mix in the soy sauce, water, honey, and black pepper, and stir to form a smooth sauce. Return the eggplant to the Instant Pot; lock the lid. Press Manual and cook on

High Pressure for 5 minutes. Use the —Quick Release‖ method to vent the steam, then open the lid. 3. Serve.

Nutrition Facts

Calories 268, Total Fat 7.9g, Saturated Fat 5.9g, Cholesterol 0mg, Sodium 546mg, Total Carbohydrate 42.4g, Dietary Fiber 20.8g, Total Sugars 22.3g, Protein 6.9g

Cottage Chesses Peanut Stir-Fry

(Prep time: 10 min |Cooking Time: 10 min | serve: 2)

Ingredients

2 tablespoons vegetable oil

½ cup frozen stir-fry vegetables

¼ teaspoon ginger powder

Salt and pepper to taste

1 egg, beaten

¼ cup corn-starch

1 cup cottage cheese, drained and cubed

1/8 cup peanut sauce

1 tablespoon chopped peanuts

Instructions

Turn Instant Pot to Sauté mode once the "Hot" sign
displays vegetable oil and add vegetables until tender.
Mix in the ginger powder, and season with salt and

pepper. Remove vegetables from the pot, and set them aside. Place the egg in a bowl. In a separate bowl, mix the corn-starch, salt, and pepper. Dip cottage cheese cubes first in the egg, then the corn-starch mixture to coat.

Heat the remaining oil in the Instant Pot to Sauté mode and cook the coated cottage cheese 5 minutes or golden brown. Stir in the peanut sauce and peanuts. Continue to cook and stir until sauce has thickened and cottage cheese is well-coated. Serve with vegetables.

Nutrition Facts

Calories 394, Total Fat 25.5g, Saturated Fat 5.8g, Cholesterol 91mg, Sodium 899mg, Total Carbohydrate 17.4g, Dietary Fiber 2.2g, Total Sugars 8.9g, Protein 22.8g

Keto Pierogies Using Fathead Dough

Delicious Keto Pierogies made with Fathead Dough are the perfect low carb pierogi substitute! You can fill them with almost anything but this version uses cheesy cauliflower puree!

Prep Time: 20 minutes Cook Time: 17 minutes Total Time: 37 minutes Servings: 12

Ingredients

For the Keto Pierogi Dough:

2   cups super fine blanched almond flour

2 cups shredded full fat mozzarella cheese 1/4 cup butter

1 large egg

1 large egg yolk For the Keto Pierogi Filling:

1 cup Cheesy Cauliflower Puree, chilled or at room temperature 1 tsp dried onion flakes

To cook and serve:

1/2 cup thinly sliced yellow onions 3 Tbsp butter

salt and pepper to taste

Instructions

To make the Keto Pierogi Dough:

Combine the mozzarella cheese and butter in a medium bowl and microwave for 1 minute. Stir, then microwave another minute. Stir until fully combined and cool for 2 minutes. Stir in the egg and egg yolk until combined.

Add the almond flour and stir with a large spoon until combined. Turn out dough onto smooth surface (or parchment paper) and knead until a semi-stretchy dough is formed. (if the dough is too wet, add a tablespoon or more of almond flour until workable)

To make the Keto Pierogies:

Divide the dough into 12 equally sized balls. Press each ball into a disk about 4 inches around.

Combine the Cheesy Cauliflower Puree and dried onion flakes and mix well. Place about 1.5 tablespoons of room temperature Cheesy Cauliflower Puree onto one half of each disk, leaving a half inch border to seal. Fold the dough over the filling and pinch to seal. Chill 10 minutes or freeze until ready to use (if cooking from frozen, thaw first).

To cook and serve the Keto Pierogi:

Melt the butter in a large saute pan over medium heat.

Add the onions and cook for 5 minutes or until soft and translucent. Add 6 of the pierogies to the pan and cook for 3 minutes per side or until the dough has turned golden brown. Remove and set aside.

Cook the remaining 6 pierogies the same way. Serve warm with the onions and butter over the top.

Nutrition Info

Serving Size: 2 Pierogies with 1 Tbsp onions in butter
Calories: 503

Fat: 46g Carbohydrates: 7g net Protein: 20g

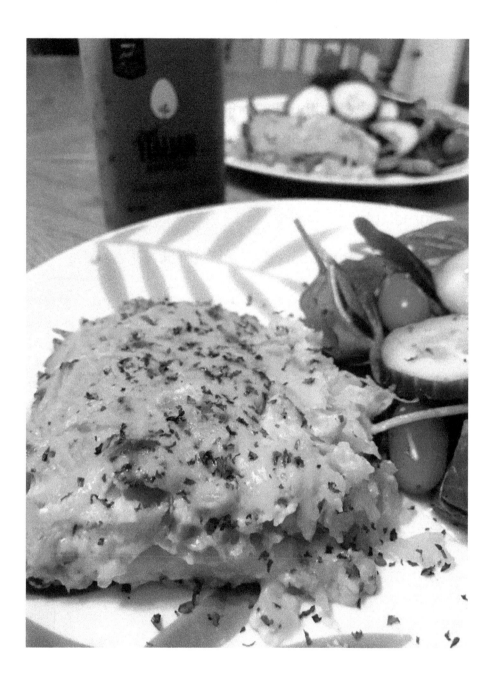

Eggplant Gratin With Feta Cheese

Prep Time: 15 minutes Cook Time: 40 minutes Total Time: 55 minutes Servings: 6

Ingredients

2   eggplants , sliced ½ inch thick

½ cup Crème Fraîche

½ cup half and half

3   oz Feta cheese crumbled 1 tsp thyme leaves chopped 1 tbsp chives chopes

4-5 basil leaves

¾ cup Gruyere cheese grated

½ cup tomato sauce 3 tbsp olive oil

salt, pepper to taste

Instructions

Preheat the oven to 375 F.

Place sliced eggplant on a parchment lined baking pan (you might need to use 2 pans). Sprinkle both sides with salt and pepper and brush with olive oil. Bake for about 20 minutes until eggplant is tender. Meanwhile, in a small saucepan, combine Crème fraîche, half and half and Feta cheese. Bring to a boil and remove from the heat. Stir in thyme and chives and set aside.

In 2.5-quart baking dish or gratin dish spread tomato sauce to cover the bottom. Place eggplant slices. They can slightly overlap each other. Spread tomato sauce once again and sprinkle with ¼ cup of Gruyere cheese. Scatter 1-2 torn basil leaves over the sauce. Continue layering with remaining eggplant, sauce and basil. Finish with pouring over the cream and Feta sauce and sprinkling with the remaining Gruyere cheese.

Bake for 15-20 minutes until bubbly and the top is browned. Serve warm.

Nutrition Info

Calories: 302kcal Carbohydrates: 14g Protein: 9.4g

Fat: 24.3g

Saturated Fat: 11.7g Cholesterol: 34mg Sodium: 335mg Potassium: 534mg Fiber: 6.8g

Sugar: 7.7g

Calcium: 220mg

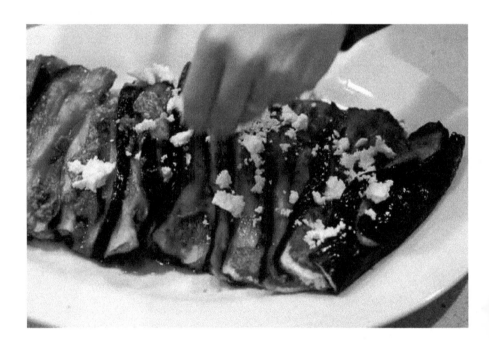

Roasted Caprese Tomatoes with Basil dressing

Roasted Caprese tomatoes with creamy mozzarella and fresh basil is a delicious and easy side dish recipe and perfect as a Summer appetizer served with crusty bread.

Prep Time: 5 minutes Cook Time: 30 minutes Total Time: 35 minutes Servings: 4

Ingredients

6 ripe tomatoes

1   tablespoon olive oil

2   tablespoons Balsamic vinegar salt & pepper to taste

6 thin slices Mozzarella 6 basil leaves for the dressing

small handful fresh basil 1 garlic clove

juice of 1/2 lemon

2 tablespoons olive oil salt and pepper to taste

Instructions

Pre-heat the oven to 180°C/350°F.

Halve the tomatoes and place on a non-stick baking sheet, cut side up. Drizzle over the olive oil and Balsamic and season with salt and pepper then top the 4 bottom halves with the mozzarella and basil leaves. Add the tops of the tomatoes. Roast for 20-25 minutes until the skins are blistered and the tomatoes are soft.

To make the dressing, blitz all the ingredients in a small food processor until the basil is finely chopped. Serve the tomatoes drizzled with the dressing with crusty bread.

Nutrition Info

Calories: 198kcal Carbohydrates: 9g Protein: 8g

Fat: 15g Saturated Fat: 4g

Cholesterol: 16mg Sodium: 166mg Potassium: 467mg
Fiber: 2g

Sugar: 6g

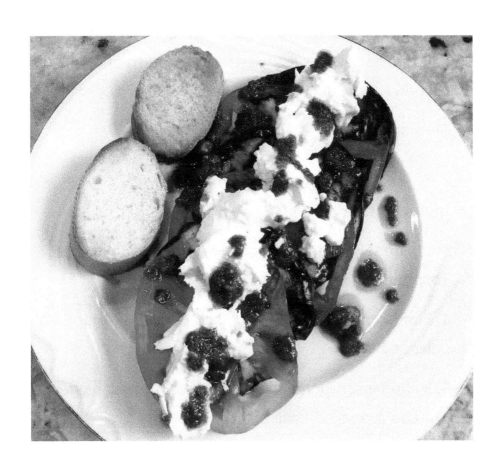

Cheesy Low Carb Cauliflower Risotto in Creamy Pesto Sauce

This versatile low carb side dish recipe perfectly mimics a classic risotto but is made with cauliflower and smothered in a cheesy pesto sauce. Keto and Atkins friendly.

Servings: Four 1 cup serving

Ingredients

4 cups finely chopped (or grated) raw cauliflower 2 Tbsp butter

1/2 tsp kosher salt 1/8 tsp black pepper 1/4 tsp garlic powder

1/3 cup Mascarpone cheese 2 Tbsp Parmesan cheese 1/4 cup prepared basil pesto

Instructions

Combine the cauliflower, butter, salt, pepper, and garlic powder in a microwave safe bowl. Microwave on high for six minutes – or until the cauliflower is tender and done to your liking. Add the mascarpone cheese and microwave on high for 2 more minutes.

Add the parmesan cheese and stir until fully blended and creamy. Cool for 2 minutes (so you don't cook the pesto when you add it and lose the green color.)

Stir in the basil pesto and serve warm.

Nutrition Info

225 calories 21g fat

4g net carbs 6g protein

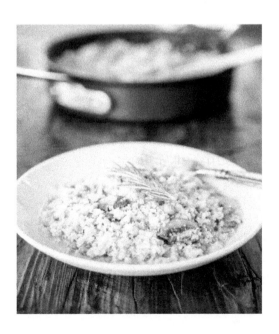

Vegetarian Greek Collard Wraps

Servingss 4 servings

Ingredients

Tzatziki Sauce

1 cup full-fat plain Greek yogurt 1 teaspoon garlic powder

1 tablespoon white vinegar 2 tablespoons olive oil

2.5 ounces cucumber, seeded and grated (¼-whole) 2 tablespoons minced fresh dill

Salt and pepper to taste

The Wrap

4 large collard green leaves, washed

1 medium cucumber, julienned

½ medium red bell pepper, julienned

½ cup purple onion, diced

8 whole kalamata olives, halved

½ block feta, cut into 4 (1-inch thick) strips (4-oz) 4 large cherry tomatoes, halved

Instructions

Mix all of the ingredients for the tzatziki sauce together and also store in the fridge. Be sure to squeeze all of the water out of the cucumber after you grate it. Prepare collard green wraps by washing leaves well and trimming the fibrous stem from each leaf. Spread 2 tablespoons of tzatziki onto the center of each wrap and smooth the sauce out. Layer the cucumber, pepper, onion, olives, feta and tomatoes in the center of the wrap. I've shown them spread out in a line to display each ingredient, but when assembling these wraps it works best to keep all of the ingredients close and toward the center of the leaf. Imagine piling them high rather than spreading them out! Fold as you would a burrito, folding in each side toward the center and the folding the rounded end over the filling and roll. Slice in halves and serve with any leftover tzatziki or wrap in plastic for a quick lunchtime meal!

Nutrition Info

165.34 Calories

11.25 g Fat 7.36g Net Carbs 6.98g Protein

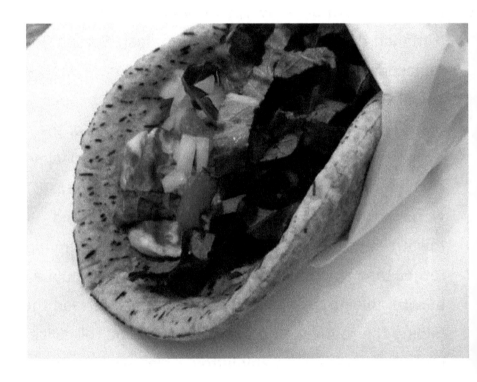

Sweets

Berry Muffins

Prep time: 15 min Cooking Time: 30 min serve: 2

Ingredients

½ cup coconut flour 1 tablespoon rolled oats

1 tablespoon honey ½ teaspoon baking powder

¼ teaspoon ground cinnamon ¼ cup coconut milk

1 egg, beaten 1 tablespoon coconut oil

½ cup fresh blueberries 1 cup water

Instructions

In a medium-size bowl, combine coconut flour, oats, honey, baking powder, and cinnamon. Stir in milk, egg, and oil. Continue stirring until the mixture is well blended. Fold in the blueberries. Spoon the mixture into the muffin cups 2/3 full.

Pour 1 cup water into the Instant Pot. Place the trivet inside. Place the muffin cups on the rack or pan.

Secure the lid and set the Pressure Release valve to Sealing. Press the Pressure Cook or Manual button and set the cook time to 20 minutes.

When the Instant Pot beeps, allow the pressure to release naturally for 10 minutes, then carefully switch the Pressure Release valve to Venting. When fully released, open the lid. Carefully remove the muffins.

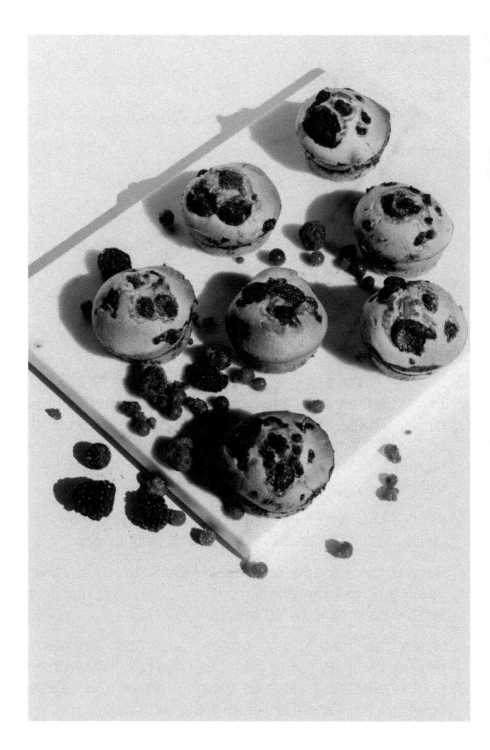

Eggplant Walnut Muffins

Prep time: 15 min Cooking Time: 30 min serve: 2

Ingredients

½ cup coconut flour

¼ teaspoon salt

¼ teaspoon ground nutmeg

¼ teaspoon baking soda

¼ teaspoon baking powder

1 egg

½ tablespoon honey

1 tablespoon coconut oil

½ cup grated eggplant

1 tablespoon walnut

1 cup water

Instructions

Mix coconut flour, salt, nutmeg, baking soda, and baking powder in a mixing bowl.

Beat egg, honey, and coconut oil together in a large bowl. Fold eggplant and walnut into egg mixture until evenly mixed. Stir flour mixture into the wet mixture to make a batter. Divide batter into muffin cups to about 2/3 full.

Pour 1 cup water into the Instant Pot. Place the trivet inside. Place the muffin cups on the rack or pan.

Secure the lid and set the Pressure Release valve to Sealing. Press the Pressure Cook or Manual button and set the cook time to 20 minutes.

When the Instant Pot beeps, allow the pressure to release naturally for 10 minutes, then carefully switch the Pressure Release valve to Venting. When fully released, open the lid. Carefully remove the muffins.

Nutrition Facts

Calories 71, Total Fat 4.8g, Saturated Fat 3.6g, Cholesterol 41mg, Sodium 248mg, Total Carbohydrate

5.7g, Dietary Fiber 0.9g , Total Sugars 4g, Protein 1.9g

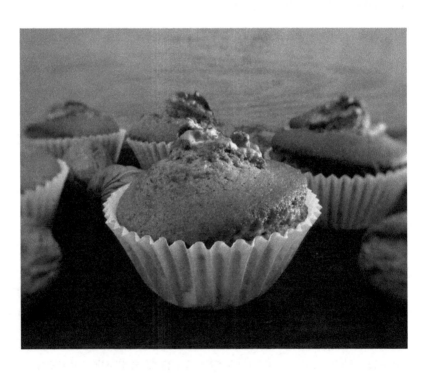

Strawberry Corn Muffins

Prep time: 15 min Cooking Time: 30 min serve: 2

Ingredients

½ cup chia seed flour

1/8 cup yellow cornmeal

½ tablespoon honey

1/8 teaspoon salt

1/8 teaspoons baking powder

1/8 teaspoon baking soda

¼ tablespoon olive oil

½ teaspoon vanilla extract

1 egg

½ cup buttermilk

¼ cup fresh strawberries

1 cup water

Instructions

In a large bowl, combine chia seed flour, cornmeal, honey, salt, baking powder and baking soda. In a separate bowl, beat together olive oil, vanilla and egg.

Stir egg mixture into dry ingredients alternating with the buttermilk just until moistened.

Gently fold in the Strawberries. Spoon batter into prepared muffin tins. Pour 1 cup water into the Instant

Pot. Place the trivet inside. Place the muffin cups on the rack or pan.

Secure the lid and set the Pressure Release valve to Sealing. Press the Pressure Cook or Manual button and set the cook time to 20 minutes.

When the Instant Pot beeps, allow the pressure to release naturally for 10 minutes, then carefully switch the Pressure Release valve to Venting. When fully released, open the lid. Carefully remove the muffins.

Nutrition Facts

Calories 80, Total Fat 2.9g , Saturated Fat 0.8g, Cholesterol 42mg , Sodium 194mg, Total Carbohydrate

10.6g, Dietary Fiber 0.8g , Total Sugars 4.8g, Protein 3.2g

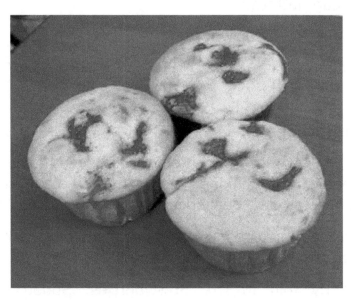

Raspberry Crumble Bars

Raspberry Crumble Bars are easy, healthy, keto, low-carb, paleo, and vegan breakfast bars. A delicious gluten-free dessert with only 7 grams of net carbs per slice.

Prep Time: 20 mins Cook Time: 30 mins Total Time: 50 mins

Ingredients

BOTTOM LAYER

2 cups Almond Flour

2 cups unsweetened desiccated coconut 1/2 cup Coconut Flour

4 tablespoons Coconut oil melted

6 tablespoons sugar free syrup or honey or maple syrup 2 tablespoons Vanilla extract

1/4 teaspoon salt

8-10 tablespoons Water

TOP LAYER

1cups Frozen Raspberries 1/4 cup Water

1/2 cup Chia seeds

1/4 cup sugar free syrup or maple syrup or honey 1 teaspoon Vanilla extract

1 cup Coconut chips 1/3 cup Almond Flour

1/2 cup unsweetened desiccated coconut

3 tablespoons sugar free natural liquid sweetener or honey or maple syrup

2 tablespoons Coconut oil 1/4 teaspoon salt

Instructions

Preheat oven to 350°F (180°C).

Prepare an 8-inch square baking tray covered with parchment paper. Set aside.

BOTTOM LAYER

In a food processor with the S blade attachment, add the almond meal, desiccated coconut, coconut flour, honey, salt, coconut oil and vanilla, and water (start with 8 tbsp). Process until it gets crumbly and all the ingredients are coming together. If too crumbly - it means it does not form a dough ball when firmly pressed within your hands - add 2 extra tablespoons of water. I added 10 tablespoons of water. Always add 2 tbsp at a time and check with a small portion of the dough. If it holds well together, you added enough water.

Evenly press the batter into the prepared baking tray. I used my fingers and flattened the layer pressing with a spatula.

Using a fork, prick the base a few times on a few areas to prevent the base from popping when baking.

Bake for 15 minutes. Cooldown fully in the tray before spreading the raspberry jam on top.

RASPBERRY CHIA SEED JAM

While the bottom layer is baking, prepare the jam. In a small saucepan, add all the jam ingredients. Cook the jam under medium heat, constantly stirring to avoid burning the jam. It is ready when the raspberries are fully melted, and it forms a thick jam. It should not take more than 5-6 minutes.

Set aside in a bowl to fully cool down and thicken a little bit. You can bring the jam outside on the deck to cool down faster. It does not have to be cold, room temperature is fine.

Spread the jam onto the baked bottom layer and return in the oven for 10 minutes to set.

Remove from the oven. Set aside while you prepare the top layer.

TOP LAYER

Add all the top layer ingredients into a mixing bowl. Use your hand to combine the ingredients, rubbing the coconut oil and liquid sweetener onto the dry ingredients to create a crumbly batter. It is the messy part!

Crumble these ingredients on top of the last layer - the chia jam

- and return the tray to the oven for 10 minutes to slightly toast the coconut crumble layer.

Fully cool down for 1 hour in the pan. You can place the pan in a cooler place like outside on the deck to cool down faster. The jam must be set and at room temperature before making slices. Place the pan for 1 hour in the fridge to set the jam faster and make it easier to slice.

Keto almond flour chocolate chip cookies

Prep Time: 10 mins Cook Time: 12 mins Total Time: 22 mins

Ingredients

5.3 oz Unsalted Butter soft, roughly diced, at room temperature for 3 hours 1/2 cup Erythritol

1/4 cup Golden erythritol or more erythritol 1 large Egg at room temperature 1 teaspoon Vanilla extract

1/2 teaspoon Almond extract optional but tasty! 1/4 teaspoon Salt 1/2 teaspoon Baking soda

1/4 teaspoon Xanthan gum highly recommended, add chewy texture, avoid cookies to crumble

2 1/4 cup Almond Flour 3/4 cup Sugar-free Chocolate Chips

Instructions

Preheat oven to 180°C (375°F). Line two cookie sheets with parchment paper. Set aside.

In a large mixing bowl, beat the soft butter with erythritol and golden erythritol until light and fluffy. It should take about 45 seconds on medium speed.

Stop the beater then add in egg, vanilla, almond extract, salt, baking soda and xanthan gum. I highly recommend xanthan gum as this adds a chewy texture to your cookies and it prevent the cookies to crumble easily.

Beat again on low speed until creamy.

Beat in the almond flour on medium speed, adding the flour 1/2 cup at a time. The batter will be fluffy and more difficult to beat as it goes, that is what you want.

Stop the beater and stir in the chocolate chips with a spatula.

Storage

Refrigerate the dough for 5 minutes.

Scoop out 3 tablespoons of dough per cookie and transfer onto a baking tray, covered with a piece of parchment paper. Leave 2 thumbs space between each cookie as they will expand during baking.

Depending on the texture and shape you aim to, slightly flatten each cookie ball into a disc. For a ultra thin, wide, cookie, flat in the center, press the cookie up to 4 mm (0.2 inches). For a thicker, softer/fluffier cookie give a small pression and barely flatten the dough. Remember that the thinner the crispier they will be in the center.

Bake 10-12 minutes, in center rack, until golden on the side but still white and soft in the middle.

Remove rack from the oven and cool the cookies on the rack for 12 minutes. Don't touch them at this point, they can be fragile and crumbly.

After 12 minutes, slide a spatula under each cookies to transfer them to a cooling rack.

Cool 20 more minutes on the cooling rack before eating. Note that the cookies will get their final texture only after 4 hours on the cooling rack at room temperature. For a crispier cookie, store in the fridge! Serve with a pinch of salt to enhance the flavors.

Blueberry Milkshakes

Prep time: 05 min Cooking Time: 02 min serve: 2

Ingredients

1 cup whole fat milk

1-1/2 tablespoons maple syrup

½ teaspoon vanilla extract

2 cups blueberries

Instructions

Seat glass pitcher on the base of the Instant Pot Ace.

Add milk, maple syrup, vanilla extract and blueberries.

Secure and lock lid.

Choose the Smoothie program (1:38 minutes).

Serve immediately.

Nutrition Facts

Calories 161, Total Fat 0.5g, Saturated Fat 0g, Cholesterol 3mg, Sodium 62mg, Total Carbohydrate

33.8g, Dietary Fiber 3.5g , Total Sugars 26.5g, Protein 5.6g

Lava Cakes

Prep time:20 min Cooking Time: 30min serve: 2

Ingredients

¼ cup coconut oil

¼ cup chocolate chopped

½ cup coconut sugar

2 large eggs at room temperature

1 large egg yolk at room temperature

3 tablespoons coconut flour

Pinch salt

½ cup water

Instructions

Put the coconut oil and chocolate in a large, microwave-safe bowl. Microwave on high in 10-second bursts, stirring well after each, until a little over half of the butter has melted. Remove from the microwave oven and continue stirring until smooth.

Set the chocolate mixture aside and cool to room temperature, stirring occasionally, about 20 minutes.

Stir the coconut sugar into the chocolate mixture until smooth. Stir in the eggs one at a time, ensuring each is well incorporated before adding the next. Stir in the eggs yolk until smooth, then the flour and salt, stirring again until smooth. Divide this mixture evenly among the prepared ramekins. Do not cover the ramekins.

Pour the water in the cooker. Set a trivet in the pot, then stack the 4 ramekins on the trivet. Lock the lid onto the cooker.

Press Pressure cook on Max pressure for 8 minutes with the Keep Warm setting off.

When the machine has finished cooking, turn it off and let its pressure return to normal naturally, about 20 minutes. Unlatch the lid and open the cooker. Transfer the hot ramekins to a wire rack and cool for 15 minutes. Serve warm.

Nutrition Facts

Calories 353, Total Fat 33.6g, Saturated Fat 25.6g, Cholesterol 186mg, Sodium 158mg, Total Carbohydrate 7g, Dietary Fiber 0.1g, Total Sugars 1.9g, Protein 6.8g

Pear Cinnamon Baked Quinoa

Prep time: 05 min Cooking Time: 10 min Serve: 2

Ingredients

1/2 cup quinoa

1/3 cup coconut milk

1/4 teaspoon baking powder

1/4 teaspoon cinnamon

1/2 teaspoon vanilla

1 teaspoon honey

1/4 cup diced pears

2 cups of water

Instructions

Mix all ingredients in a bowl. Mix them well so that all quinoa is moist.

Put 2 cups of water into the Instant Pot and place the trivet on the bottom. Place the bowl in the Instant Pot and lock lid by closing the pressure valve.

Cook at High Pressure for 10 minutes with the Manual setting. When done, open the Instant Pot and let the pressure release naturally. Take the bowl out of the Instant Pot.

Serve hot.

Keto snickerdoodles

Keto snickerdoodles are easy soft keto cookies with a delicious cinnamon flavor

Prep Time: 15 mins Cook Time: 12 mins Total Time: 27 mins

Ingredients

Dry ingredients

1 1/3 cup Almond Flour

2 tablespoons Coconut Flour

1/3 cup Erythritol - erythritol or monk fruit 1/2 teaspoon Baking soda

1/2 teaspoon Xanthan gum

Liquid ingredients

1/4 cup Coconut oil or melted butter

1/4 cup Unsweetened vanilla almond milk at room temperature 1 teaspoon Vanilla essence

1 teaspoon Apple cider vinegar Cinnamon coating

2 teaspoons Ground cinnamon

3 tablespoons Erythritol - erythritol or monk fruit

Instructions

In a large mixing bowl, whisk together all the dry ingredients: almond flour, coconut flour, sweetener, baking soda, xanthan gum.

Pour the melted coconut, unsweetened almond milk (at room temperature or it will solidify the coconut oil), vanilla and apple cider vinegar.

Combine with a spoon at first, then use your hands to knead the dough and form a consistent cookie dough ball. Set aside in the bowl, at room temperature, while you prepare the cinnamon coating.

In a separate bowl, whisk together ground cinnamon and sugar- free crystal sweetener of your choice.

Shape 16 small cookie dough balls. I am using a small mechanical cookie dough scoop to make cookies of the same size and same carb count.

Roll each cookie dough balls into the cinnamon sugar-free sugar, rolling the balls in your hands to stick the coating to the balls. Place each cookie ball onto a baking tray covered with parchment paper, leaving 1 cm space between each cookie.

Flatten the snickerdoodle cookie with a spatula until the sides crack and the thickness is similar to a regular snickerdoodle cookie. These cookies won't expand while baking that is why it is important to shape/flatten them before baking.

 Repeat for the following cookies.

Bake cookies at 180°C/355°F for 15-18 minutes or until the sides are slightly golden brown, don't overbake are they won't be as soft.

Remove from the oven and cool down 5 minutes on the baking tray before transferring on a cooling rack. Slide a spatula under each cookie to gently transfer them onto a cooling rack without breaking.

The cookie are soft at first when out of the oven, they will harden and reach their best texture at room temperature, about 1 hour cool down required.

Nutrition Info

Calories 76 Calories from Fat 43 Fat 4.8g Carbohydrates 2.2g Fiber 0.8g Sugar 0.5g1% Protein 1.2g

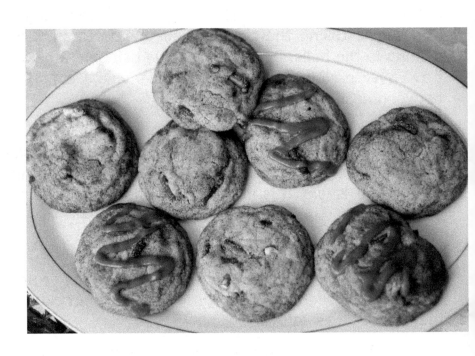

Low carb shortbread cookies with almond flour

Those low carb shortbread cookies with almond flour are easy 5 ingredients healthy shortbread cookies perfect for the holidays.

Prep Time: 10 mins Cook Time: 10 mins Total Time: 20 mins

Ingredients

1 1/3 cup Almond Flour 1/4 cup erythritol

1/4 cup Soft Unsalted Butter at room temperature for 3 hours

1/2 teaspoon Vanilla essence

1/8 teaspoon salt Chocolate decoration - optional

1 oz Sugar-free Chocolate Chips 1/2 teaspoon Coconut oil

Instructions

Preheat oven to 356 F (180C).

Cover a baking sheet with parchment paper. Set aside.

Mix all of the ingredients together until it forms a cookie crumble - about 1 minute. You can use a stand mixer with a hook attachment or an electric mixer.

Gather the cookie crumble with your hands to form a cookie ball.

Refrigerate 10 minutes in a bowl.

Remove from the fridge, scoop 1 teaspoon of dough onto the prepared baking sheet leaving a thumb space between each cookie. You can also roll the dough in your hands and form balls. Then use a fork to slightly flatten the cookie.

Bake your shortbread cookies for 8 -11 minutes or until they start to be golden brown on the top.

Remove from the oven and cool down for 10 minutes on the baking sheet before transferring them to a cooling cookie rack to cool completely before decorating.

Add the sugar free chocolate and coconut oil into a saucepan. Under medium heat, stir and melt the chocolate.

Use a scoop to drizzle a bit of chocolate on some (or all) cookies.

Store the cookies in a cookie jar up to 3 weeks.

Nutrition Info

Calories 81 Calories from Fat 68 Fat 7.5g Carbohydrates 1.9g Fiber 1g Sugar 0.4g Protein 2.1g

Sweet snowballs

Prep:20 mins Cook: 5 mins Plus chilling Easy Makes 16

Ingredients

400g white chocolate, broken into pieces

100g rich tea biscuit

50g white Malteser

50g mini marshmallow

50g dried cranberries

50g cake crumbs (we used shop-bought Madeira cake) 3 tbsp golden syrup

100g desiccated coconut

edible glitter (optional)

Directions:

Melt the chocolate in a bowl over a pan of simmering water. Meanwhile, crush the biscuits and Maltesers in a large bowl with a rolling pin.

Add mini marshmallows, dried cranberries and cake crumbs, then the chocolate and golden syrup. Mix well. Tip desiccated coconut onto a plate. Drop large spoonfuls of mixture onto the plate, roll them around, coating in coconut, and shape into balls. Place on a baking tray and chill for 30 mins before serving. Sprinkle with edible glitter if you like.

Rainbow cookies

Prep: 25 mins - 30 mins Cook:15 mins Easy Makes 22

Ingredients

175g softened butter

50g golden caster sugar

50g icing sugar

2 egg yolks

2 tsp vanilla extract

300g plain flour

zest and juice 1 orange

140g icing sugar, sifted

sprinkles, to decorate

Directions:

Heat oven to 200C/180C fan/gas 6. Mix the butter, sugars, egg yolks and vanilla with a wooden spoon until creamy, then mix in the flour in 2 batches. Stir in the orange zest. Roll the dough into about 22 walnut-size balls and sit on baking sheets. Bake for 15 mins until golden, then leave to cool.

Meanwhile, mix the icing sugar with enough orange juice to make a thick, runny icing. Dip each biscuit half into the icing, then straight into the sprinkles. Dry on a wire rack.

Lightning Source UK Ltd.
Milton Keynes UK
UKHW021403070521
383306UK00005B/125